Kimberly Coy

Covid Baby

D1719331

Bumblebee Books
London

A CIP catalogue record for this title is
available from the British Library.

ISBN: 978-1-83934-612-5

Bumblebee Books is an imprint of
Olympia Publishers.

First Published in 2022

Bumblebee Books

Tallis House
2 Tallis Street
London
EC4Y 0AB

Printed in Great Britain

www.olympiapublishers.com

Dedication

I dedicate this book to all of the families who have taken the best care of their covid babies.

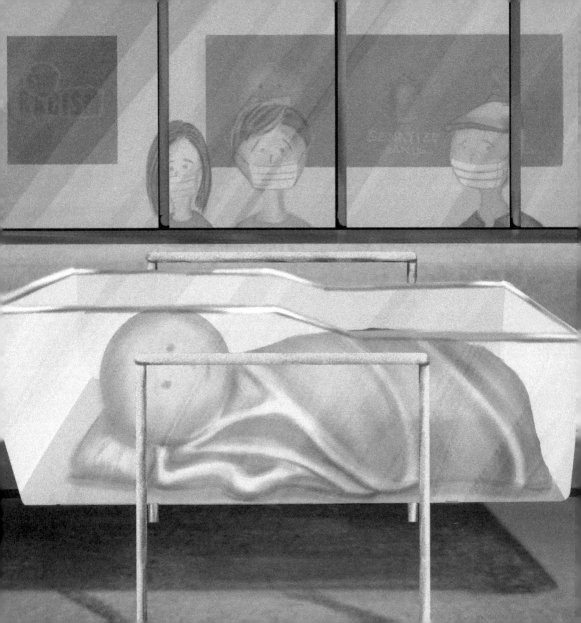

Covid Baby was born during the covid 19 pandemic. It was a time of sickness, fear, and change.

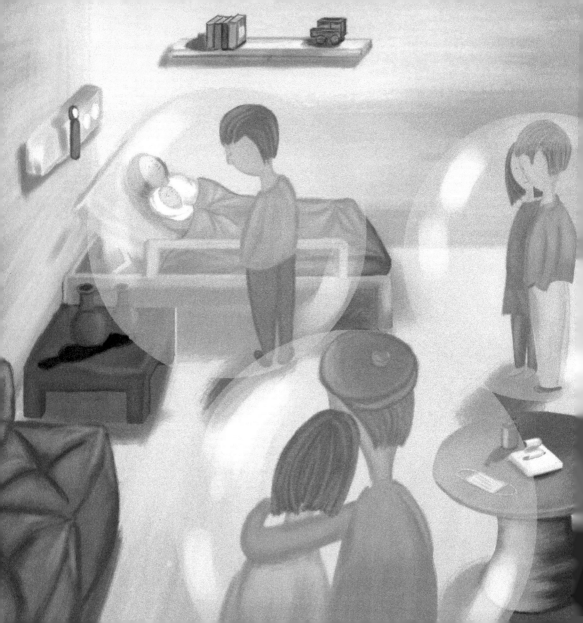

Covid Baby was born in a bubble of love.

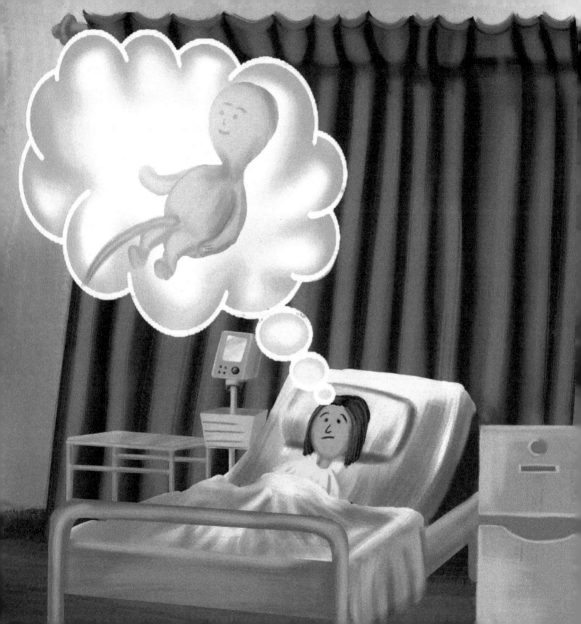

Covid Baby's mom was in the hospital for a long time. She was lonely, and thought of Covid Baby all of the time.

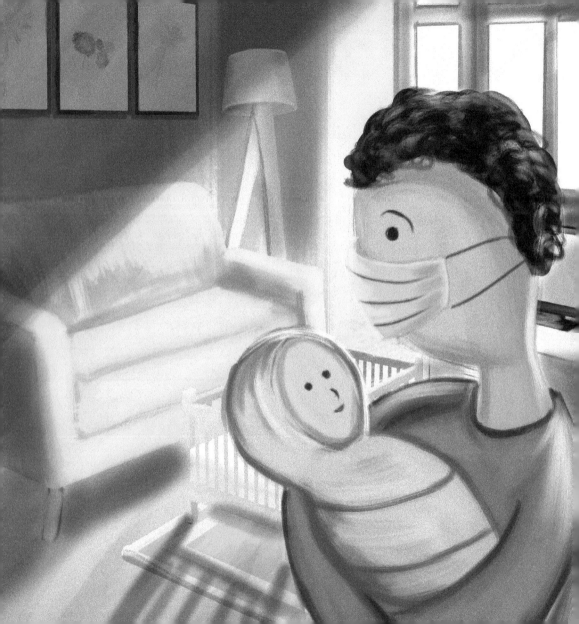

When Covid Baby was born, Dad got to come and hold her!

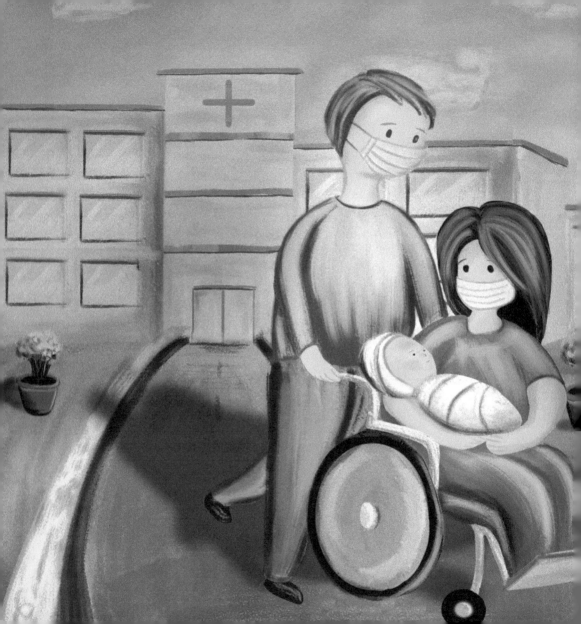

Covid Baby's mom and dad were so excited to take her home.

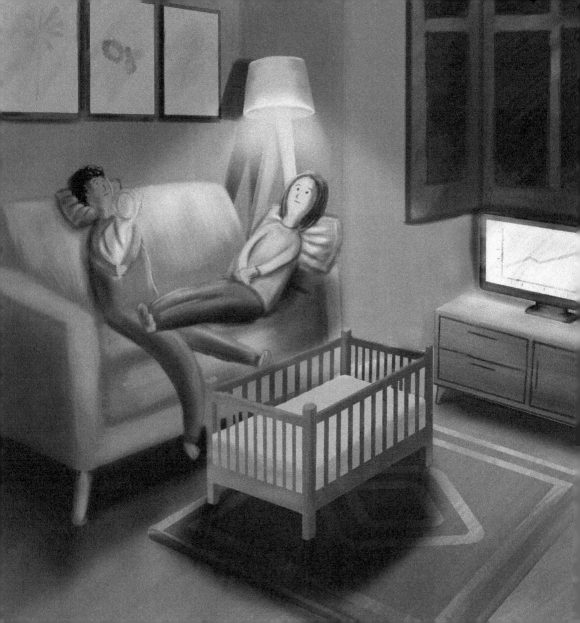

Covid Baby takes all naps only in laps.

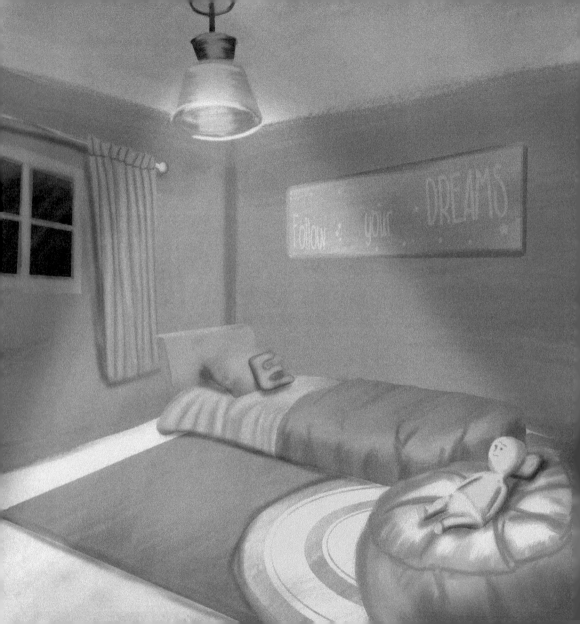

Covid Baby's best friends are in her home.

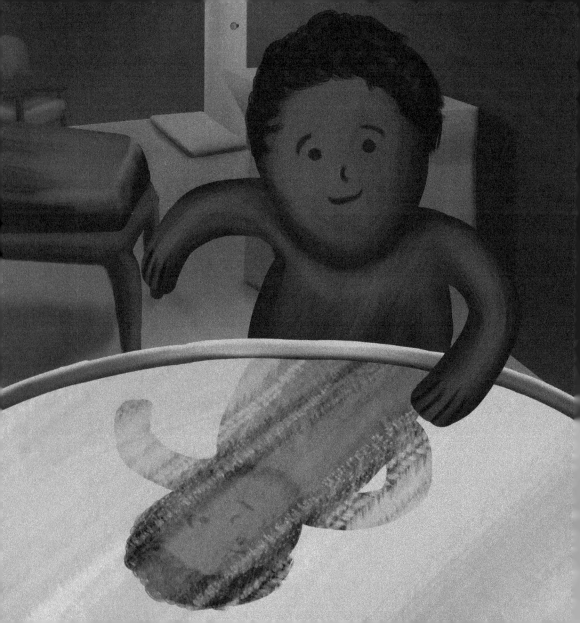

Covid Baby's best friends are in her mirror.

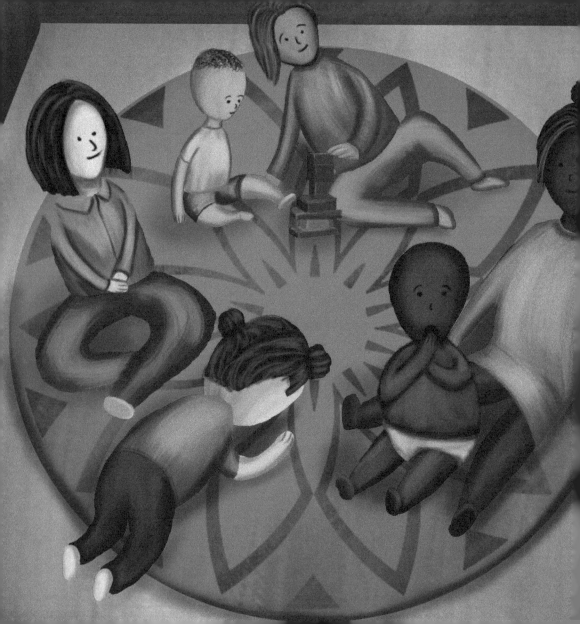

Covid Baby could not go to baby groups.

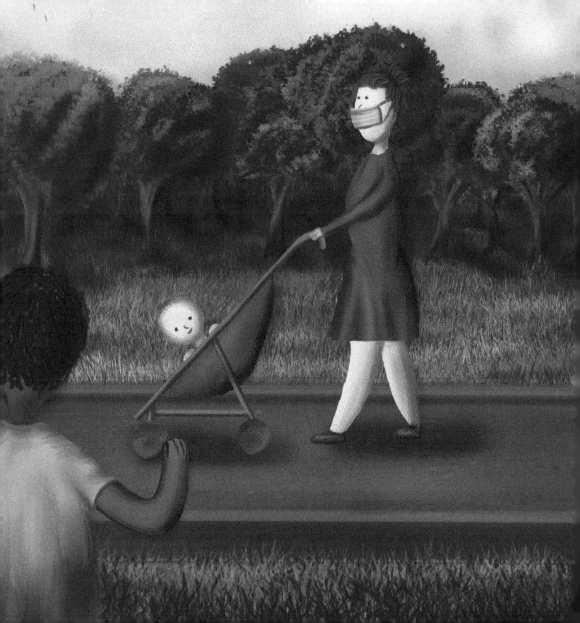

There were many baby activities
Covid Baby could not do.

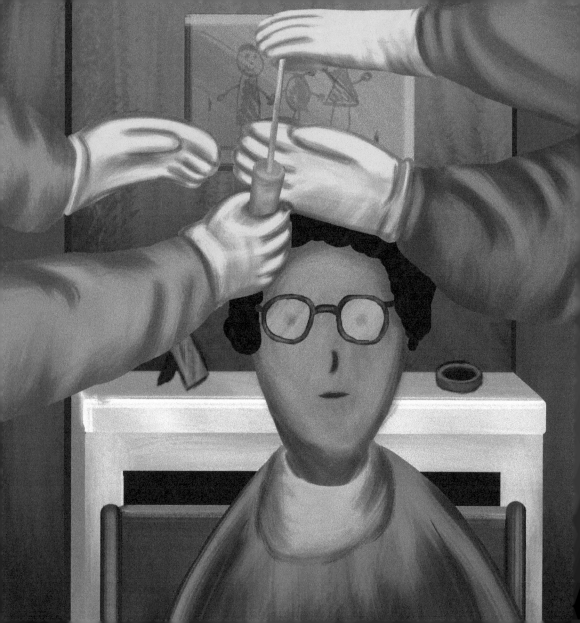

Covid Baby's grandparents took many covid tests to keep her safe.

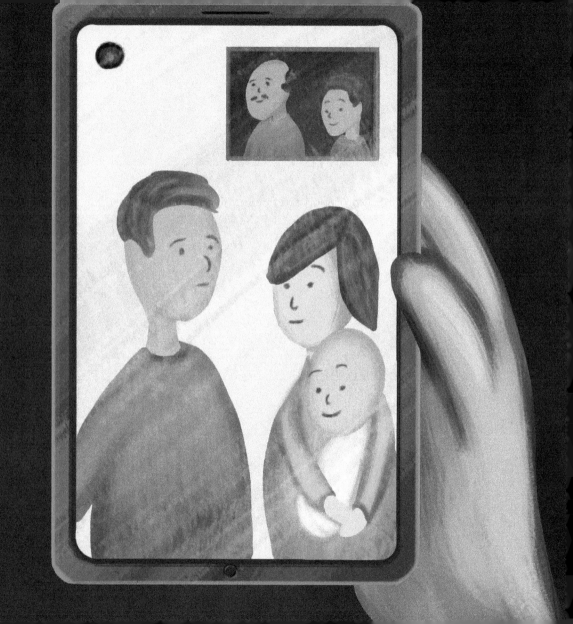

Even first holidays were quite for
Covid Baby.

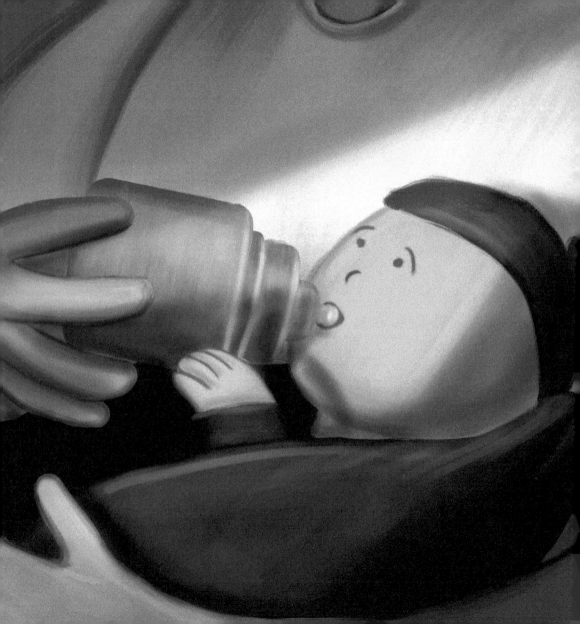

Covid Baby could not eat solid foods for a long time because an allergy could send her to the hospital, and hospitals were not safe for covid babies because there was not a vaccine for her yet.

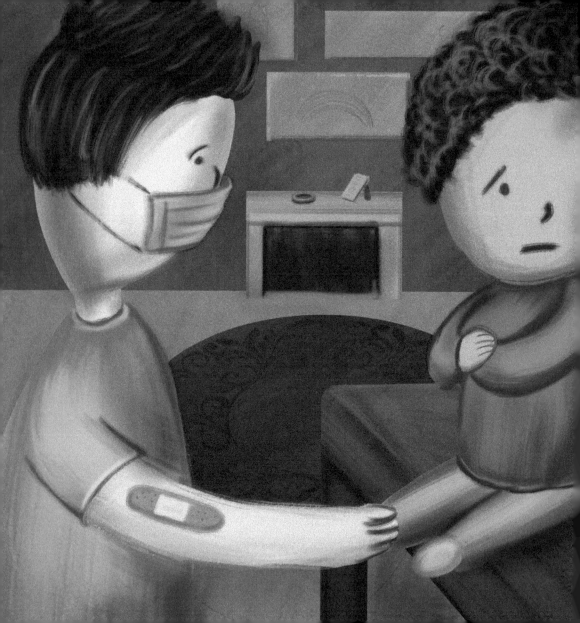

Only people with vaccinations could meet her.

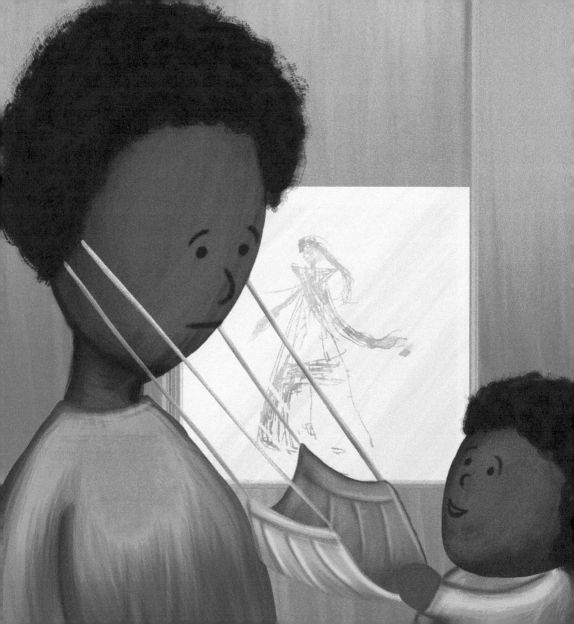

Covid Baby knew face masks were just right for people outside her home.

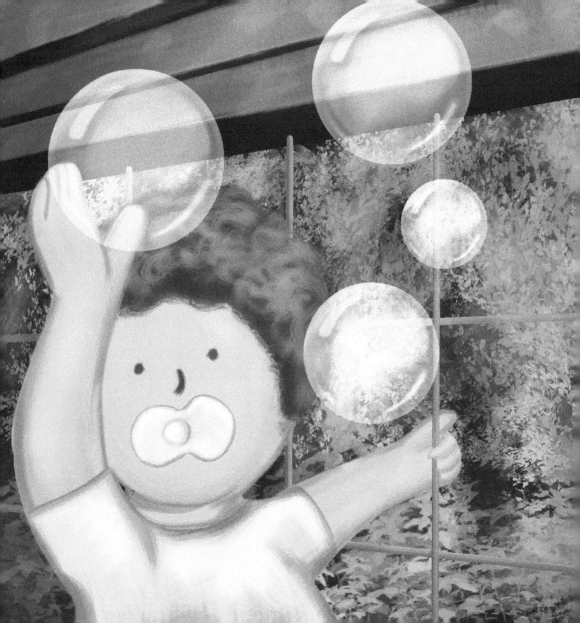

When Covid Baby is old enough she will get the vaccine too and explore her new world.

About the Author

Kimberly Coy teaches in the Kremen School of Education and Human Development at the California State University in Fresno California. She has been lucky enough to read thousands of children's books to students during her career. With this first children's book she has returned to the love of sharing stories.

Acknowledgements

Thank you to my family, loves of my life.

CPSIA information can be obtained
at www.ICGtesting.com
Printed in the USA
BVHW091651270522
638317BV00015B/370

9 781839 346125